K.Z. MATSON

INVINCIBLE HEALTH

Simple Strategies To Optimize Your Health, Fitness, Energy and Mood

This book was professionally typeset on Reedsy.
Find out more at reedsy.com

Contents

1

Introduction

High-functioning people don't focus on problems; they focus on solutions and prevention. Being proactive and taking responsibility for our health is the key to living a long, productive, and serviceable life.

Years ago, I had an 84-year-old client who was still working five hours a day in the construction trades. He was vigorous and quick-witted. I asked him what his secret was. He replied; "I stay away from doctors and hospitals." He went on to share his diet and fitness regimen which included whole foods, some herbal supplementation, vitamins and minerals, and daily calisthenics.

Certainly, modern medicine is crucial to treating and dealing with critical and acute health issues. However, today's MDs receive woefully little training in diet and nutrition.

In addition, much of our food supply is either depleted of its nutrient content and is even contaminated with pesticides, herbicides hormones, and antibiotics to name a few. We must jealously guard what we put into our bodies if we want them to function well and remain resilient and strong into our 80s.

2

Supplementation

The importance of supplementation in maintaining optimal health and well-being, setting the tone for the rest of the chapter.

Supplementation plays a vital role in supporting our overall health and well-being. In today's fast-paced world, it can be challenging to get all the nutrients we need from diet alone. This is where supplements come in, offering a convenient way to fill in the gaps and support our bodies' functions. By understanding the different types of supplements available and how they can benefit us, we can take proactive steps towards optimizing our health and vitality for the long term.

Different Types of Supplements - The various types of supplements available, including vitamins, minerals, herbs, and other dietary supplements, highlighting their potential benefits and considerations.

There is a vast array of supplements available in the market today, each offering unique benefits for our health and well-being. Vitamins, such as Vitamin C and Vitamin D, play essential roles in supporting our immune system, maintaining strong bones, and promoting overall health. Minerals like iron, calcium, and magnesium are crucial for various bodily functions, including blood circulation, bone health, and muscle function.

Herbal supplements, derived from plants and botanicals, have been used for centuries in traditional medicine to enhance health and treat various ailments. Popular herbs like turmeric, ginseng, and echinacea are known for their anti-inflammatory, antioxidant, and immune-boosting properties. Additionally, omega-3 fatty acids, sourced from fish oil or plant-based sources like flaxseed, offer numerous cardiovascular and cognitive benefits.

Other dietary supplements, such as probiotics, prebiotics, and collagen peptides, target specific areas of health, such as gut health, digestion, and skin elasticity. Understanding the potential benefits and considerations of each type of supplement is essential for selecting the right ones to support your individual health needs. Always prioritize quality, safety, and consult with healthcare professionals before adding any new supplements to your regimen.

How to choose the right supplements for your individual needs, emphasizing the importance of quality, safety, and consulting with healthcare professionals

When navigating the supplement landscape, it's essential to prioritize quality and safety. Look for reputable brands with third-party testing to ensure purity and potency. Consult a healthcare professional to determine which supplements are best suited for your individual needs, taking into account factors like age, gender, diet, and any existing health conditions. Keep in mind that supplements are intended to complement a healthy diet, not replace it. Be cautious of extravagant health claims and always read the labels carefully to understand the ingredients and proper dosage. Remember, your health is priceless, so invest wisely in supplements that support your well-being.

**** Exploring the Benefits of Supplements****

Vitamins play a crucial role in our overall well-being, supporting various bodily functions and promoting optimal health. From Vitamin A for vision to Vitamin D for bone health, these essential nutrients help regulate important processes in the body.

Minerals are another key component in maintaining our health. Minerals like calcium, potassium, and iron are essential for proper muscle function, nerve transmission, and oxygen transport in the blood. Ensuring an adequate intake of minerals is vital for our overall vitality.

Clean water is often overlooked as a vital supplement for our health. Staying hydrated is essential for proper digestion, nutrient absorption, and temperature regulation. Drinking enough water daily can help flush out toxins, support healthy skin, and boost energy levels. Remember, staying hydrated is a simple yet powerful way to support your body's overall health and vitality.

**** - The role of supplements in supporting overall health and vitality.****

Supplements play a crucial role in supporting our overall health and vitality. In today's fast-paced world, it's not always easy to get all the essential nutrients our bodies need from food alone. This is where supplements come in, providing a convenient way to bridge the gap and ensure we are meeting our nutritional requirements.

By incorporating supplements into our daily routine, we are able to support our immune system, improve energy levels, and enhance our overall well-being. Whether it's a vitamin to boost our immunity, a mineral to support bone health, or an herbal supplement to reduce stress, each supplement plays a unique role in helping us maintain optimal health.

Moreover, supplements can act as a safety net, providing additional support during times of increased stress, illness, or when our diet may be lacking in essential nutrients. They offer a simple and effective way to fill in any nutrient gaps and support our bodies in functioning at their best.

In essence, supplements are like a secret weapon in our health arsenal, helping us to thrive and feel our best every day. By understanding their role and incorporating them thoughtfully into our routine, we can take proactive steps towards enhancing our overall health and vitality.

**** - Highlighting how supplements can help fill in nutrient gaps in our diets.****

When we strive to maintain our well-being, ensuring that we receive all the necessary nutrients plays a crucial role. Our diets may sometimes fall short in providing us with the essential vitamins and minerals needed for optimal health. This is where supplements come in handy as a convenient way to bridge the gap and support our overall well-being.

Supplements offer a convenient means of obtaining nutrients that may be lacking in our daily meals. Even with the most balanced diet, it can be challenging to meet all our nutritional needs solely through food. By incorporating supplements into our routine, we can ensure that we are getting all the vital nutrients our bodies require to function at their best.

Whether it's busy schedules, dietary restrictions, or specific health conditions that prevent us from getting all the nutrients we need, supplements can play a valuable role in filling those gaps. They offer a simple and effective way to boost our nutrient intake and support our overall health and vitality.

By taking supplements that fill in these nutrient gaps, we can help safeguard our health and well-being in the long run. It's important to remember that supplements are meant to complement a healthy diet and lifestyle, not replace them. They serve as a valuable tool in our wellness toolkit, providing added support to help us thrive and feel our best.

**** - Common reasons why people turn to supplementation for added support.****

Many individuals turn to supplementation for added support due to various reasons. One common motivation is the desire to address specific health concerns such as low energy levels, weakened immune system, or poor skin health. Supplements offer a convenient and targeted way to provide the body with essential nutrients that may be lacking in one's diet.

Furthermore, some people use supplements as a preventive measure to support overall well-being and optimize their health. With busy lifestyles and hectic schedules, it can be challenging to consistently consume a well-balanced diet that meets all nutritional needs. In such cases, supplements can serve as a reliable backup to ensure the body receives adequate vitamins, minerals, and other vital nutrients.

Moreover, certain life stages or circumstances may increase the need for supplementation. For example, pregnant women often require additional folic acid and iron to support their own health and the healthy development of their baby. Similarly, older adults may benefit from specific supplements to promote bone health or cognitive function as they age.

Additionally, athletes and individuals who engage in intense physical activity may turn to supplements to enhance performance, support muscle recovery, or address nutrient losses during training. The targeted nature of supplements can help these individuals meet their unique nutritional needs and optimize their athletic performance.

Overall, the reasons for turning to supplementation are diverse and multifaceted, reflecting the individual health goals, needs, and circumstances of each person. By understanding these motivations, individuals can make informed choices about incorporating supplements into their wellness routine to support their overall health and vitality.

** Understanding Different Types of Supplements**

Sure, here is the detailed, engaging section on "Understanding Different Types of Supplements":

Exploring the world of supplements opens up a treasure trove of possibilities for enhancing your health and well-being. Vitamins, minerals, and herbal supplements each bring their unique benefits to the table, offering a diverse range of options to support your body's needs.

Vitamins play a crucial role in numerous bodily functions, from bolstering immunity to promoting healthy skin and hair. Whether you're looking to up your intake of vitamin C for its immune-boosting properties or vitamin D to support bone health, these essential nutrients can help bridge the gap between dietary deficiencies and optimal health.

Minerals are another cornerstone of supplement options, with key players like calcium, magnesium, and iron playing vital roles in maintaining overall wellness. Calcium, for example, is essential for strong bones and teeth, while magnesium aids in muscle function and relaxation. Incorporating these minerals into your supplement regimen can help fortify your body's foundation for long-term health.

Herbal supplements offer a natural alternative to traditional vitamins and minerals, tapping into the power of plants to support various health concerns. From chamomile for calming nerves to echinacea for immune support, these botanical remedies provide a holistic approach to well-being that resonates with many individuals seeking gentler, plant-based solutions.

Navigating the realm of supplements can feel overwhelming at first, but understanding the different types available allows you to tailor your approach to meet your specific health goals. Whether you're looking to boost your energy levels, support your immune system, or address a specific health issue, selecting the right combination of vitamins, minerals, and herbal supplements can empower you to take charge of your health in a personalized and effective way.

** - The various categories of supplements such as vitamins, minerals, and herbal supplements.**

Vitamins are essential for various bodily functions. They act as catalysts for reactions in the body and play a crucial role in maintaining overall health. Some common vitamins include Vitamin A, B-complex vitamins, Vitamin C, Vitamin D, and Vitamin E. These vitamins can be found in a variety of foods, but supplementation may be necessary for individuals who have specific dietary restrictions or deficiencies.

Minerals are another important category of supplements that are vital for proper bodily functions. Minerals such as calcium, magnesium, zinc, iron, and potassium are crucial for maintaining the balance of fluids in the body and supporting various physiological processes. Mineral supplements can help ensure that individuals meet their daily requirements, especially if their diet lacks these essential nutrients.

Herbal supplements have gained popularity for their potential health benefits derived from plant-based sources. These supplements often contain compounds that are believed to have medicinal properties and can support overall well-being. Some common herbal supplements include turmeric, echinacea, ginseng, and ginger. While herbal supplements can offer natural remedies, it's essential to research and consult with a healthcare provider to ensure their safety and effectiveness.

Understanding the various categories of supplements, including vitamins, minerals, and herbal supplements, can help individuals make informed choices about their health and well-being. By incorporating these supplements into a balanced diet and healthy lifestyle, individuals can support their overall health and vitality.

**** - How to choose high-quality supplements and avoid potential pitfalls.****

When selecting supplements, it's crucial to prioritize quality over quantity. Look for reputable brands that have been tested for safety and efficacy. Consider factors such as third-party certifications, transparency in ingredient sourcing, and absence of harmful additives like fillers or artificial colors. Reading customer reviews and seeking recommendations from healthcare professionals can offer valuable insights into the reliability of a supplement. Be wary of exaggerated health claims or promises of quick fixes – remember that supplements are meant to complement a well-rounded diet, not replace it. Always check the dosage instructions and potential side effects before starting a new supplement regimen, and listen to your body's response as you introduce new products. By taking a thoughtful and informed approach to selecting supplements, you can optimize their benefits while minimizing any potential risks or drawbacks.

**** - The importance of consulting with a healthcare provider before starting a new supplement regimen.****

It's important to consult with a healthcare provider before starting a new supplement regimen. Your doctor or a qualified healthcare professional can offer valuable insights and guidance to ensure that the supplements you choose are safe and appropriate for your individual needs. They can help you understand any potential interactions with medications you may be taking and provide personalized recommendations based on factors like your age, health status, and dietary habits. By seeking professional advice before incorporating new supplements into your routine, you can make informed decisions that support your overall health and well-being.

**** Tips for Incorporating Supplements Into Your Routine****

When incorporating supplements into your daily routine, it's essential to approach it with a sense of mindfulness and care. One key tip is to start slowly and introduce one supplement at a time. This allows you to gauge how your body responds and identify any potential adverse reactions.

Another helpful tip is to set a consistent schedule for taking your supplements. Whether it's with breakfast, lunch, or dinner, establishing a routine can help ensure you don't forget to take them.

Consider organizing your supplements in a pill organizer or setting reminders on your phone to stay on track with your regimen. This simple strategy can make a significant difference in maintaining consistency and adherence.

It's also crucial to store your supplements properly in a cool, dry place away from direct sunlight. This helps preserve their potency and effectiveness over time.

Remember to listen to your body and be mindful of any changes or improvements you notice while taking supplements. Consulting with a healthcare provider if you have any concerns or questions is always a wise decision to ensure you're getting the most out of your supplement regimen.

**** - Practical advice on how to integrate supplements into your daily life.****

When it comes to integrating supplements into your daily routine, simplicity is key. Start by establishing a consistent schedule for taking your supplements, whether it's first thing in the morning, with a meal, or before bed. Consider setting a daily reminder on your phone or placing your supplements in a visible location to help you remember to take them.

To make it easier to remember which supplements to take and when, consider organizing them in a pill organizer or creating a chart to track your daily intake. This can help ensure that you are taking the correct dosages and staying on top of your supplement routine.

Incorporating supplements into your routine can also be more enjoyable by trying different forms of supplements, such as gummies, powders, or capsules. Find what works best for you and makes the experience more enjoyable.

Lastly, be patient and allow time for the supplements to take effect. Results may not be immediate, so give your body time to adjust and respond to the added support. Consistency is key, so stick to your routine and monitor how you feel over time to assess the impact of the supplements on your overall health and well-being.

**** - Ways to track your supplement intake and monitor their effects on your health.****

One effective way to track your supplement intake is by creating a daily or weekly journal where you can record which supplements you have taken and at what dosage. This can help you stay organized and ensure that you are consistently taking your supplements as recommended.

Another useful method is to set reminders on your phone or computer to take your supplements at the same time each day. This can help establish a routine and make it easier to remember to take them.

Monitoring the effects of your supplements on your health is essential for determining their efficacy. Keep track of any changes you notice in your energy levels, mood, digestion, or other areas of your health. This information can help you and your healthcare provider assess whether the supplements are benefiting you.

It is also important to be patient when it comes to seeing the benefits of supplementation. Some supplements may take time to show noticeable effects, so consistency in taking them as directed is key. Trust the process and continue to monitor how you feel over time to gauge their impact on your overall well-being.

**** - The importance of consistency and patience when it comes to seeing the benefits of supplementation.****

Consistency and patience are key when it comes to reaping the benefits of supplementation. It's essential to understand that supplements work best when taken consistently over time. Think of it as a gradual process of nourishing and supporting your body's needs. Rome wasn't built in a day, and neither is optimal health. By staying committed to your supplement routine, you give your body the best chance to utilize these additional nutrients effectively.

It's important to have realistic expectations and not expect overnight transformations. Just like a plant needs time to grow and blossom, your body needs time to absorb and benefit from the supplements you're providing it. Trust in the process and have faith that your efforts will pay off in the long run.

Consistency doesn't mean perfection. If you happen to miss a dose here and there or forget to take your supplements for a day, don't fret. It's about the overall pattern of regular intake that matters most. Be gentle with yourself and pick up where you left off without guilt or self-criticism.

Patience is a virtue, especially when it comes to health and well-being. Remember, change takes time, and the effects of supplementation may not be immediate. Allow your body the time it needs to respond and adapt to the nutrients you're providing it. Trust that your consistent efforts will lead to positive outcomes in the long term.

In a world of instant gratification, practicing patience with your health journey can be a powerful and empowering choice. Celebrate the small victories along the way and acknowledge the progress you're making, even if it's not always visible on the surface. Your commitment to consistency and patience will ultimately yield lasting benefits for your overall health and vitality.

3

Nourishing Your Body with the Right Foods

**** Building a Foundation of Nutrient-Rich Foods****

Get ready to revamp your eating habits by focusing on nutrient-rich foods. It's time for an oil change - ditch the bad oils and make room for the good ones. Opt for nutrient-dense foods that pack a powerful punch of vitamins and minerals. Don't forget to include fiber in your meals for optimal digestion and overall health. When choosing meats and produce, go organic for cleaner and more nutritious options. Next time you're at the grocery store, stick to the perimeter aisles where you'll find fresh, whole foods to nourish your body from the inside out.

**** Understanding the Impact of Processed Foods****

When it comes to processed foods, it's important to be aware of the impact they can have on your health. These convenient and often tasty options may come with a hidden cost. Processed foods are typically loaded with added sugars, unhealthy fats, and artificial additives that can wreak havoc on your body over time.

Consuming a diet high in processed foods has been linked to various health concerns, including obesity, heart disease, and diabetes. These foods are often stripped of their natural nutrients during processing and then fortified with synthetic vitamins and minerals, which may not be as beneficial as the real deal.

Reading food labels is crucial when trying to navigate the world of processed foods. Look out for ingredients like high-fructose corn syrup, hydrogenated oils, and artificial flavors or colors. Opting for whole, unprocessed foods whenever possible is a simple yet powerful way to protect your health and well-being.

By being mindful of your consumption of processed foods and making a conscious effort to prioritize whole, nutrient-dense options, you can take a significant step towards improving your overall health and vitality.

Incorporating Healthy Eating Habits into Your Lifestyle

Strategies for meal planning, grocery shopping, and preparing meals ahead of time can make a significant impact on your overall health and well-being. By taking the time to plan out your meals for the week, you can ensure that you have nutritious options readily available and reduce the temptation to rely on processed or convenience foods. Consider batch cooking on the weekends to prepare meals in advance, making it easier to grab a healthy option during busy weekdays.

Mindful eating practices can help you cultivate a more positive relationship with food and listen to your body's hunger and fullness cues. Take the time to savor and appreciate each bite, focusing on the flavors and textures of your food. Avoid distractions such as eating in front of the TV or computer, and instead, create a peaceful environment where you can fully enjoy your meals.

Embrace a flexible approach to nutrition that allows for occasional indulgences while prioritizing nourishing foods. Remember that a balanced diet is about consistency over perfection, so don't be too hard on yourself if you have a treat now and then. Strive for progress, not perfection, and be kind to yourself as you make healthier choices for your body.

By incorporating these healthy eating habits into your lifestyle, you can create a sustainable and enjoyable approach to nourishing your body and fueling your overall well-being.

4

Moving Your Body for Increased Vitality

In this chapter, we delve deeper into the myriad ways you can move your body to enhance your vitality and overall well-being. Movement is a fundamental aspect of human existence, and the benefits of regular physical activity extend far beyond mere physical fitness. By incorporating a variety of movement practices into your daily routine, you can cultivate a profound connection to your body, increase your energy levels, and promote optimal health.

1. **Aerobic Exercise for Cardiovascular Health:** Aerobic exercise, also known as cardiovascular exercise, is essential for maintaining a healthy heart and circulatory system. Activities such as running, cycling, dancing, and swimming elevate your heart rate, improve lung capacity, and enhance your body's ability to transport oxygen to your muscles. Regular aerobic exercise not only strengthens your cardiovascular system but also boosts your mood, reduces stress levels, and supports cognitive function. Aim for a combi-

nation of moderate-intensity and high-intensity cardiovascular exercises to maximize the benefits for your heart health and overall vitality.

2. **Strength Training for Muscle Health:** Building and maintaining muscle mass is crucial for overall health and vitality, especially as we age. Strength training exercises, such as weightlifting, bodyweight exercises, and resistance band workouts, help increase muscle strength, endurance, and power. In addition to enhancing physical performance, strength training can boost metabolism, support weight management, and improve bone density. By incorporating a variety of resistance exercises into your fitness routine, you can sculpt a strong, resilient body that supports you in all areas of life.

3. **Flexibility and Mobility for Joint Health:** Flexibility and mobility are key components of physical fitness that often get overlooked. Stretching exercises, yoga, Pilates, and mobility drills help improve joint range of motion, reduce muscular tension, and enhance overall flexibility. Maintaining optimal flexibility is essential for preventing injuries, improving posture, and supporting a full range of movement in daily activities. Regular stretching sessions can also promote relaxation, reduce stress levels, and increase body awareness, fostering a deeper sense of connection to your physical form.

4. **Mindful Movement Practices for Mind-Body Connection:** Mindful movement practices, such as tai chi, qigong, and yoga, offer a unique opportunity to cultivate a deeper connection between your mind and body. These practices emphasize breath awareness, mindfulness, and gentle, intentional movements that promote relaxation, stress reduction, and emotional balance. By engaging in mindful movement, you can enhance your proprioception, improve coordination, and heighten your awareness of subtle

body sensations. This mind-body connection extends beyond the physical realm, influencing your emotional well-being, mental clarity, and overall sense of vitality.

5. **Integrating Holistic Movement Practices for Comprehensive Well-being:** To experience holistic vitality, consider integrating a variety of movement practices into your daily life. Explore activities that challenge different aspects of your physical fitness, such as balance, agility, coordination, and endurance. Engage in nature-based movement practices like hiking, trail running, or outdoor yoga to connect with the natural world and rejuvenate your spirit. Experiment with new movement modalities, such as dance, martial arts, or calisthenics, to keep your workouts dynamic and engaging. By embracing a diverse range of movement practices, you can nurture your body, mind, and spirit, and cultivate a lasting sense of vitality and well-being.

In conclusion, movement is a vital aspect of human existence that contributes to our overall vitality and well-being. By incorporating a variety of movement practices into your daily routine, you can enhance your physical fitness, mental clarity, emotional balance, and spiritual connection. Find joy in moving your body, embrace the diversity of movement modalities available to you, and discover the profound transformation that occurs when you prioritize movement for increased vitality. Embrace the power of movement to nourish your body, invigorate your spirit, and live a life filled with energy, passion, and purpose.

5

The Importance of Quality Sleep

In the hustle and bustle of modern life, where deadlines loom large and responsibilities seem never-ending, the simple act of getting a good night's sleep can often be overlooked. Yet, the truth remains undeniable - quality sleep is a cornerstone of our health and well-being, playing a profound role in every aspect of our lives.

As we delve deeper into the realm of sleep, we uncover the intricate mechanisms that govern this essential process. Our bodies follow a delicate dance of sleep stages, cycling through periods of light sleep, deep sleep, and rapid eye movement (REM) sleep, each playing a unique role in our physical and mental restoration. It is during these stages that our brain clears out waste products, consolidates memories, and promotes cellular repair and growth throughout our body.

The impact of sleep extends far beyond simple rest and rejuvenation; it intertwines with nearly every system in our bodies. One of the key players in this symphony is the circadian rhythm, our internal body clock that regulates our sleep-wake cycle. Disruptions to this delicate balance, such as shift work or jet lag, can wreak havoc on our health, leading to a host of negative consequences, including increased inflammation, metabolic dysfunction, and cognitive impairment.

Furthermore, the connection between sleep and mental health is a profound one. Adequate sleep is essential for emotional regulation, cognitive function, and overall mental well-being. Studies have shown that sleep deprivation can exacerbate symptoms of anxiety and depression, while getting enough rest can improve mood, enhance creativity, and bolster our resilience in the face of life's challenges.

The benefits of quality sleep extend to our physical health as well. Chronic sleep deprivation has been linked to an increased risk of obesity, cardiovascular disease, and diabetes. During sleep, our bodies release hormones that regulate appetite and metabolism, meaning that a lack of sleep can disrupt these crucial processes, leading to weight gain and metabolic dysfunction over time.

To truly embrace the importance of quality sleep, we must recognize it as a pillar of our health alongside nutrition and exercise. Establishing healthy sleep habits, such as maintaining a consistent sleep schedule, creating a relaxing bedtime routine, and optimizing our sleep environment, can pave the way for a more vibrant and fulfilling life.

So, as you prepare to drift off into the realm of dreams tonight, remember the profound impact that quality sleep has on your health and well-being. Cherish this time of rest and rejuvenation, for it is within the peaceful embrace of sleep that your body and mind find the nourishment they need to thrive.

6

Managing Stress for Overall Well-being

In today's modern society, stress has become a pervasive force that impacts individuals from all walks of life. The fast-paced nature of our world, coupled with the constant demands of work, relationships, and daily responsibilities, can easily lead to feelings of overwhelm and tension. It is essential to recognize the detrimental effects of chronic stress on both our physical and mental health and take proactive steps to manage and alleviate it for overall well-being.

One of the most potent tools for combating stress is the ancient practice of meditation. Meditation offers a gateway to inner peace and tranquility by quieting the mind and allowing a deeper connection to our inner self. Research has shown that regular meditation practice can reduce stress, anxiety, and even symptoms of depression. By dedicating just a few minutes each day to mindfulness meditation or guided visualization, individuals can cultivate a sense of calm and emotional balance amidst life's challenges.

In addition to meditation, the power of focused breathing techniques cannot be overstated in stress management. Deep breathing exercises, such as diaphragmatic breathing or the 4-7-8 technique, can help shift the body from a state of fight-or-flight to a state of relaxation. By consciously engaging in deep, slow breaths, individuals can activate the parasympathetic nervous system, leading to a decrease in heart rate, blood pressure, and cortisol levels. This simple yet profound practice can be done anywhere, at any time, making it an accessible tool for immediate stress relief.

Cold therapy, a growing trend in wellness circles, is another effective method for stress reduction and overall well-being. Exposure to cold temperatures through cold showers, ice baths, or cryotherapy has been found to activate the body's natural healing processes, increase circulation, and boost mood-enhancing neurotransmitters. Cold therapy can act as a potent stress reliever by stimulating the release of endorphins, which are known as the body's natural painkillers and mood elevators. Embracing the invigorating power of cold therapy can provide a refreshing and revitalizing experience for both the body and mind.

Nature, with its inherent beauty and serenity, offers a sanctuary for stress relief and rejuvenation. Engaging in practices like forest bathing, or Shinrin-yoku in Japanese, involves immersing oneself in the sights, sounds, and scents of the natural world to promote relaxation and well-being. Research has shown that spending time in nature can reduce levels of the stress hormone cortisol, lower blood pressure, and improve mood and cognitive function. The healing power of nature acts as a grounding force, reconnecting individuals with the rhythms of the earth and providing a sense of calm and restoration amidst the chaos of daily life.

Sound therapy, an ancient healing modality that utilizes sound vibrations to bring about relaxation and balance, is gaining popularity as a stress management tool in modern times. Listening to calming music, nature sounds, or binaural beats can help regulate brainwave patterns, induce a state of deep relaxation, and alleviate stress and anxiety. Sound therapy can be used in various forms, such as sound baths, gong therapy, or even simply listening to soothing melodies to create a peaceful environment. By immersing oneself in the harmonious frequencies of sound, individuals can experience a profound sense of calm and rejuvenation for overall well-being.

Self-care is a fundamental pillar of stress management and plays a crucial role in maintaining balance and resilience in the face of life's challenges. Engaging in activities that nurture the mind, body, and spirit, such as exercise, creative pursuits, or spending quality time with loved ones, can replenish energy reserves and promote emotional well-being. Setting boundaries and prioritizing self-care is essential in preventing burnout and maintaining a healthy work-life balance. By honoring one's needs and practicing self-compassion, individuals can cultivate a sense of inner strength and empowerment to navigate stressors effectively.

Understanding the intricate relationship between stress and health is key to developing effective coping strategies and promoting overall well-being. Chronic stress can have far-reaching consequences on the body, leading to a range of physical and mental health issues, including cardiovascular disease, immune system suppression, and mood disorders. By recognizing the signs of stress and implementing holistic approaches to manage it, individuals can safeguard their health and enhance their quality of life.

In conclusion, managing stress is an ongoing journey that requires a multifaceted approach encompassing mindfulness practices, breathing techniques, cold therapy, nature immersion, sound therapy, self-care activities, and stress awareness. By integrating these tools into daily life, individuals can cultivate resilience, emotional balance, and a sense of inner peace. Prioritizing mental and physical well-being through intentional self-care practices is a vital investment in overall health and longevity. Embrace the wisdom of ancient healing practices and modern stress management techniques to foster a life of vitality and harmony.

7

Cultivating a Positive Mindset

**** Embracing Gratitude and Positivity****

Garbage in, Garbage out. Jealousy guard not only what goes in your mouth but also what enters your being through your eyes and ears. Speak well to yourself - positive self-talk. Your self-talk is your soul. We all talk to ourselves even though we are unaware of it. Get a Power Statement. Give yourself positive atta-boys or atta-girls affirming what you did well and do well.

**** Overcoming Limiting Beliefs and Negative Self-Talk****

Identifying and challenging the negative thoughts that hold you back is a crucial step toward fostering a positive mindset. Often, our limiting beliefs and negative self-talk stem from fears and insecurities that have been ingrained over time. It's important to recognize these patterns and actively work towards reframing them in a more constructive light.

Cultivating self-compassion and self-acceptance is a powerful tool in overcoming limiting beliefs. Instead of harshly criticizing ourselves for perceived shortcomings or failures, we can choose to approach ourselves with kindness and understanding. By practicing self-compassion, we can create a supportive inner dialogue that encourages growth and resilience.

Negative self-talk can often amplify challenges and setbacks, making them seem insurmountable. By reframing challenges as opportunities for growth, we can shift our perspective and approach difficulties with a sense of empowerment. Viewing setbacks as learning experiences helps us build resilience and develop a mindset that is focused on progress rather than perfection.

** Cultivating Optimism and Resilience**

Developing a resilient mindset in the face of adversity is a key factor in maintaining a positive outlook on life. Resilience allows us to bounce back from setbacks and challenges, viewing them as opportunities for growth rather than insurmountable obstacles. By cultivating optimism, we can create a brighter future for ourselves, focusing on the possibilities rather than dwelling on the negatives. Building mental strength through mindfulness and meditation can help us stay grounded and centered, even amid chaos. These practices enable us to tap into our inner reserves of strength and resilience, empowering us to face whatever life throws our way with grace and courage.

8

Creating a Supportive Environment for Health

**** Setting Up Your Physical Space ****

Organizing your home and work environment for optimal health is key to creating a space that supports your well-being. Clearing clutter and creating designated areas for different activities can help reduce stress and promote a sense of calm. Incorporating elements of nature, such as plants and natural lighting, can enhance the overall ambiance of your space and positively impact your mood. Consider decluttering your space regularly and adding personal touches that bring you joy and comfort, making your environment a sanctuary for relaxation and rejuvenation.

**** Cultivating Supportive Relationships ****

Building meaningful relationships that support your health journey is a key ingredient in creating a fulfilling and nourishing life. Surround yourself with individuals who uplift and empower you, those who share your vision for well-being. These supportive relationships can provide the encouragement and motivation needed to stay committed to your health goals. Remember, it's not just about the quantity of relationships, but the quality of the connections you have. Cultivate relationships that bring out the best in you and where there is mutual respect and understanding.

Establishing healthy boundaries in your relationships is essential for maintaining a sense of balance and emotional well-being. Learn to communicate your needs openly and assertively, while also respecting the boundaries of others. By fostering a culture of respect and understanding in your relationships, you create a safe and nurturing environment for personal growth and self-care.

Building a network of friends and family who share your values and beliefs about health can provide a strong support system for your well-being journey. Whether it's cooking nutritious meals together, engaging in physical activities, or simply offering emotional support, having a tribe of like-minded individuals can make a world of difference in staying committed to your health goals. Surround yourself with positivity and encouragement, and watch how your relationships can be a powerful force in helping you thrive in all aspects of your life.

**** Engaging in Community and Social Activities ****

Participating in community and social activities is a wonderful way to enhance your overall well-being and create a sense of connection with others. Whether you choose to join a local fitness class, volunteer at a community event, or join a club that aligns with your interests, engaging in social activities can bring joy and fulfillment to your life.

Being part of a supportive community can provide you with a sense of belonging and purpose, as well as opportunities to meet new people and make lasting connections. By participating in group activities, you can share your passions with like-minded individuals and expand your social circle in a fun and enriching environment.

Community and social activities also offer a chance to break out of your routine, try new things, and explore different interests. Whether you enjoy hiking, dancing, painting, or sports, there are countless opportunities to engage in activities that bring you joy and fulfillment.

Additionally, volunteering in your community is a wonderful way to give back and make a positive impact on the world around you. By lending a helping hand to those in need, you can create a sense of purpose and contribute to the well-being of others.

Overall, engaging in community and social activities can enrich your life in many ways. It can boost your mood, improve your social skills, and provide a sense of connection and belonging that is essential for overall health and well-being. So go out there, explore new opportunities, and immerse yourself in the vibrant tapestry of community life.

9

Sustaining Long-Term Health Habits

**** Establishing Consistent Routines:****

Establishing consistent routines is key when it comes to maintaining long-term health. By incorporating regular habits into our daily lives, we create a structure that supports our well-being and sets us up for success. These routines help us stay on track with healthy behaviors, making it easier to prioritize our physical and mental health.

One important aspect of establishing consistent routines is setting realistic goals. By breaking down larger health objectives into smaller, manageable steps, we can make steady progress over time. This approach not only makes our goals more achievable but also allows us to celebrate our victories along the way.

Monitoring our progress is another crucial component of maintaining consistent routines. By keeping track of our habits and behaviors, we can identify patterns, assess our successes and challenges, and make adjustments as needed. This self-awareness helps us stay accountable and motivated to continue working toward our long-term health goals.

Incorporating daily practices into our routines can also support our overall well-being. Whether it's scheduling time for physical activity, preparing nutritious meals, or incorporating stress-relief techniques, these habits can have a positive impact on our health. By making these practices a regular part of our lives, we create a foundation for sustainable health and vitality.

In essence, establishing consistent routines is about creating a lifestyle that prioritizes our health and well-being. By building habits that support our physical, emotional, and mental wellness, we can set ourselves up for long-term success and fulfillment.

** - The importance of establishing regular habits and routines in maintaining long-term health.**

Establishing regular habits and routines is crucial for maintaining long-term health. Consistency breeds success when it comes to our well-being. By incorporating healthy practices into our daily lives, we create a foundation for sustainable lifestyle changes. Small, manageable steps gradually lead to significant improvements in our overall health and vitality. Whether it's starting the day with a nutritious breakfast, engaging in regular physical activity, or practicing stress-relief techniques, every positive habit contributes to our well-being. Setting realistic goals and monitoring our progress helps us stay on track and adjust our routines as needed. By building a solid framework of healthy habits, we pave the way for long-term health and wellness.

** - Strategies for creating sustainable lifestyle changes, such as setting realistic goals and monitoring progress.**

Creating sustainable lifestyle changes requires a thoughtful approach that focuses on setting realistic goals and tracking progress. By establishing habits and routines that align with your long-term health goals, you can build a strong foundation for overall well-being. Start by identifying specific areas where you want to make improvements, whether it's increasing physical activity, adopting a healthier diet, or managing stress more effectively.

Setting achievable goals is key to staying motivated and seeing tangible results. Break down larger objectives into smaller, manageable steps that you can work towards consistently. This could involve committing to a certain number of workouts per week, incorporating more fruits and vegetables into your meals, or dedicating time each day for relaxation techniques. By setting realistic targets, you create a roadmap for success that is both challenging and attainable.

Monitoring your progress is essential in staying on track and adjusting your strategies as needed. Keep a journal or use a tracking app to record your daily habits, feelings, and achievements. This can help you identify patterns, celebrate successes, and pinpoint areas that may need more attention. Reflect on your progress regularly and celebrate each milestone, no matter how small it may seem. By acknowledging your efforts and progress, you can stay motivated and continue making positive changes toward a healthier lifestyle.

**** –Daily practices that can contribute to overall well-being, including exercise, nutrition, and stress management techniques.****

Engaging in daily practices that prioritize your overall well-being is essential for sustaining long-term health habits. By incorporating simple yet impactful activities into your routine, you can nurture your body and mind, setting the foundation for a healthier and more balanced lifestyle.

Begin your day with a nourishing breakfast to fuel your body for the challenges ahead. Enjoy a mix of protein, healthy fats, and carbohydrates to provide sustained energy throughout the morning. Incorporate nutrient-dense foods like eggs, whole grains, and fresh fruits to kickstart your day on a nutritious note.

Throughout the day, prioritize movement to keep your body active and engaged. Take short breaks to stretch or go for a brisk walk to combat sedentary habits. Physical activity not only benefits your physical health but also boosts mood and promotes mental clarity.

Incorporate mindfulness practices into your daily routine to cultivate a sense of awareness and presence. Take a few moments to focus on your breath, centering yourself in the present moment. Practice gratitude by reflecting on the positive aspects of your day, fostering a mindset of appreciation and contentment.

Prioritize stress management techniques to combat the pressures of daily life. Engage in activities that promote relaxation, such as yoga, meditation, or deep breathing exercises. Create a calming environment in your home with soothing music, aromatherapy, or a cozy reading nook to unwind and de-stress.

End your day with a restful night's sleep to recharge your body and mind. Establish a bedtime routine that promotes relaxation, such as reading a book, taking a warm bath, or practicing gentle stretches. Ensure your bedroom is a tranquil sanctuary conducive to restful sleep, free from distractions and electronic devices.

By incorporating these daily practices into your routine, you can nurture your overall well-being and support the sustainability of your long-term health habits. Take small, intentional steps each day to prioritize self-care and cultivate a balanced, healthy lifestyle that uplifts your body, mind, and spirit.

** Cultivating Mindful Awareness:**

Mindful awareness is a powerful tool that can help you sustain healthy habits and promote self-awareness in your daily life. By practicing mindfulness, you can cultivate a deeper connection to your thoughts, emotions, and physical sensations, enabling you to navigate life's challenges with more clarity and resilience.

One way to incorporate mindfulness into your routine is through meditation. Taking just a few minutes each day to sit quietly and focus on your breath can help calm the mind, reduce stress, and increase your overall sense of well-being. By bringing your attention to the present moment, you can cultivate a greater awareness of your thoughts and feelings without judgment.

In addition to formal meditation practice, you can also engage in mindfulness throughout your day by being fully present in your activities. Whether you are eating a meal, taking a walk, or having a conversation, bring your awareness to the sensations, sights, and sounds around you. By savoring the present moment and letting go of distractions, you can experience greater joy and fulfillment in your daily life.

Mindful awareness can also extend to your interactions with others. By listening attentively, observing nonverbal cues, and responding with empathy and understanding, you can deepen your connections and foster more meaningful relationships. Practicing mindfulness in your communication can help you cultivate a sense of presence and authenticity in your interactions, leading to greater harmony and connection in your social interactions.

Overall, cultivating mindful awareness is a transformative practice that can enhance your well-being and contribute to sustainable healthy habits. By bringing a sense of mindfulness to your thoughts, actions, and relationships, you can deepen your self-awareness, reduce stress, and create a foundation for living a more fulfilling and balanced life.

**** - The role of mindfulness in sustaining healthy habits and promoting self-awareness.****

Mindfulness plays a crucial role in sustaining healthy habits and fostering self-awareness. By bringing our attention to the present moment without judgment, we can better understand our thoughts, emotions, and behaviors. This heightened awareness allows us to make informed choices that align with our values and goals. Incorporating mindfulness practices into our daily routines can help us stay grounded, reduce stress, and cultivate a sense of inner peace.

One powerful way to cultivate mindfulness is through meditation. Taking a few minutes each day to sit quietly and observe our breath can significantly impact our overall well-being. By focusing on the sensations of breathing, we can anchor ourselves in the present moment and quiet the chatter of the mind. This practice not only enhances our concentration and clarity but also helps us manage stress more effectively.

Deep breathing exercises are another valuable tool for promoting mindfulness. By consciously taking slow, deep breaths, we can activate our body's relaxation response and calm the nervous system. This simple practice can be done anytime, anywhere, making it a convenient way to bring mindfulness into our busy lives. Deep breathing not only reduces anxiety and tension but also encourages us to pause and reconnect with the present moment.

Being present in the moment is a fundamental aspect of mindfulness. When we fully engage with our current experience, we can savor the richness of life and appreciate the simple joys that surround us. Whether we are eating a meal, taking a walk, or having a conversation, being fully present allows us to experience life more deeply and authentically. By letting go of distractions and focusing on the here and now, we can cultivate a sense of gratitude and contentment in our daily lives.

** - Tips for practicing mindfulness in everyday life, such as meditation, deep breathing exercises, and being present in the moment.**

Practicing mindfulness in everyday life involves bringing your full attention to the present moment without judgment. One way to do this is through meditation, which can help you cultivate a sense of calm and clarity. Find a quiet space, sit comfortably, and focus on your breath as you inhale and exhale. Notice any thoughts or sensations that arise without getting caught up in them.

Deep breathing exercises can also promote mindfulness by connecting your breath with your body and mind. Take slow, deep breaths in through your nose, feeling your belly rise, and exhale through your mouth, releasing tension and stress. Repeat this breathing technique several times to center yourself and bring awareness to the present moment.

Being present in the moment means fully engaging in whatever you are doing without distractions. Whether you are eating a meal, walking in nature, or having a conversation, try to give your complete attention to the experience. Notice the sights, sounds, smells, and tastes around you, savoring each moment without rushing or worrying about the past or future.

By incorporating these mindfulness practices into your daily routine, you can cultivate a greater sense of awareness, reduce stress, and enhance your overall well-being. Take time each day to quiet your mind, connect with your breath, and fully engage in the present moment to experience the benefits of mindfulness in your life.

**** - Explain how mindful eating and mindful movement can support long-term health goals and enhance overall quality of life.****

Mindful eating involves being fully present and attuned to your food choices and eating habits. It's about savoring each bite, paying attention to your body's hunger and fullness cues, and making conscious decisions about what and how much you eat. By practicing mindful eating, you can cultivate a healthier relationship with food and support your long-term health goals.

Similarly, mindful movement involves engaging in physical activities with awareness and intention. This could include practices like yoga, tai chi, or simply going for a walk while paying attention to your body's movements and sensations. By moving mindfully, you can enhance your physical well-being, improve your flexibility and strength, and reduce stress and tension in your body.

Both mindful eating and mindful movement can have a positive impact on your overall quality of life. They can help you develop a deeper connection to your body, improve your self-awareness, and cultivate a sense of gratitude and appreciation for the nourishment and movement your body needs. By incorporating these practices into your daily routine, you can support your long-term health goals and create a more balanced and fulfilling lifestyle.

** Building a Support Network:**

Surrounding yourself with a supportive community is crucial in maintaining healthy habits and sustaining positive lifestyle changes. A strong support network can provide encouragement, motivation, and accountability, making it easier to stay on track with your health goals. Whether it's friends, family members, or like-minded individuals who share your commitment to well-being, having a supportive community can make a significant difference in your journey toward long-term health and happiness.

By engaging with others who prioritize health and wellness, you can exchange ideas, share experiences, and learn from one another. This shared sense of purpose can inspire and empower you to stay dedicated to your health aspirations. Moreover, being part of a supportive community can help you overcome challenges and obstacles that may arise along the way. With the encouragement and guidance of those around you, navigating through setbacks becomes more manageable, and you are less likely to feel overwhelmed or discouraged.

Building a support network also creates a sense of belonging and connection, which is essential for emotional well-being. When you feel understood, accepted, and encouraged by those around you, it can positively impact your mental health and overall quality of life. Additionally, being part of a community that promotes healthy behaviors can reinforce your commitment to self-care and motivate you to prioritize your well-being.

In essence, surrounding yourself with a supportive network is a powerful asset in sustaining long-term health habits. By fostering relationships with individuals who uplift and inspire you, you can create a positive environment that nurtures your physical, mental, and emotional wellness. Together, you can encourage each other to stay focused, resilient, and committed to leading a healthy and fulfilling life.

**** - The importance of surrounding yourself with a supportive community that encourages healthy behaviors.****

Surrounding yourself with a supportive community that encourages healthy behaviors is like having a team of cheerleaders rooting for your well-being. These are the people who lift you up when you're feeling down, celebrate your successes, and keep you accountable on your health journey. Whether it's a friend who joins you for a morning workout, a family member who cooks nutritious meals with you, or a healthcare professional who provides guidance and support, having a strong support network can make all the difference in sustaining long-term health habits.

Sharing your goals and progress with others not only creates a sense of camaraderie but also motivates you to stay on track. When surrounded by individuals who prioritize health and wellness, it becomes easier to adopt positive habits and make healthier choices. Their encouragement and understanding during challenging times can help you stay committed to your well-being goals.

Building a community of like-minded individuals who value health and wellness allows for mutual inspiration and support. You can exchange ideas, share tips, and learn from each other's experiences, creating a positive environment that fosters growth and self-improvement. By surrounding yourself with a supportive community, you not only enhance your well-being but also contribute to the collective health and happiness of those around you. In this interconnected web of support, everyone thrives together, uplifting each other to lead healthier, more fulfilling lives.

**** - The benefits of seeking support from friends, family, or health professionals in maintaining motivation and accountability.****

Support from friends, family, and health professionals plays a vital role in maintaining motivation and accountability on your journey to better health. When you have a strong support system around you, you are more likely to stay on track with your health goals and make positive choices. Friends and family can offer encouragement, share experiences, and provide a listening ear when needed. Their support can help you navigate challenges and celebrate victories along the way. In addition, seeking guidance from health professionals, such as doctors, nutritionists, or personal trainers, can provide you with expert advice tailored to your specific needs. These professionals can offer valuable insights, personalized recommendations, and ongoing support to help you achieve long-term success in your health and wellness journey.

**** - How to cultivate a network of like-minded individuals who share your commitment to long-term health and well-being.****

Creating a network of like-minded individuals who share your commitment to long-term health and well-being is essential for staying motivated and accountable on your wellness journey. Surrounding yourself with supportive individuals who understand and champion your health goals can significantly impact your success in maintaining healthy habits over time. Here are some practical guidance on how to cultivate a supportive network:

Connect with like-minded individuals: Seek out groups or communities that align with your health and wellness values. This could be a local fitness group, cooking class, hiking club, or online support forum dedicated to healthy living.

Share your goals: Open up to your friends, family, or colleagues about your health objectives and the steps you are taking to achieve them. By articulating your goals out loud, you are more likely to stay committed and accountable.

Engage in activities together: Plan regular activities with your network that promote health and well-being, such as exercise classes, healthy cooking nights, or mindfulness practices. By participating in these activities together, you can strengthen your bond and encourage each other to stay on track.

Celebrate successes: Acknowledge and celebrate your achievements, big or small, with your support network. Whether it's hitting a fitness milestone, trying a new healthy recipe, or overcoming a wellness challenge, sharing your wins can boost morale and motivation within the group.

Offer support to others: Be a source of encouragement and motivation for your peers as they pursue their own health goals. By giving back and supporting others in their journey, you create a positive feedback loop of support within your network.

Stay connected: Regularly communicate and check in with your support network to maintain a sense of community and camaraderie. Whether it's through in-person meet-ups, virtual check-ins, or sharing resources and tips, staying connected can help sustain the momentum towards long-term health and well-being.

10

Embracing Joy and Purpose in Life

**** Discovering Personal Fulfillment through Service****

"Service is the rent we pay for living in this world of ours." –Spencer W. Kimball

Exploring the Connection between Joy and Purpose-

When we engage in acts of service, we often find a deep sense of fulfillment that goes beyond just helping others. It's a profound connection to our own sense of purpose and meaning in life. By extending a helping hand to those in need, we not only make a positive impact on their lives but also enrich our own in ways we may not have expected.

Finding Meaning in Giving Back to Others

There is a unique satisfaction that comes from giving back to others. Whether it's volunteering at a local charity, donating to a cause close to your heart, or simply offering a helping hand to a friend in need, the act of selflessly serving others brings a sense of purpose and fulfillment that money can't buy.

Benefits of Service for Mental and Emotional Well-being

Studies have shown that engaging in acts of service can have a profound impact on our mental and emotional well-being. By focusing our energy on helping others, we shift our perspective from our own problems and worries to the needs of those around us. This shift in focus can reduce stress, boost our mood, and increase feelings of happiness and fulfillment.

** Cultivating a Spirit of Generosity**

The power of kindness and compassion can have a profound impact on both the giver and the receiver. When we extend generosity to others, it not only uplifts their spirits but also nourishes our own souls. Small acts of kindness, whether it's a smile, a helping hand, or a thoughtful gesture, can create ripple effects of positivity that spread far and wide.

Incorporating service into our daily lives doesn't have to be overwhelming. It can be as simple as holding the door open for someone, offering a listening ear to a friend in need, or volunteering at a local charity. These acts of generosity not only brighten someone else's day but also bring a sense of fulfillment and purpose to our own lives.

When we cultivate a spirit of generosity, we develop a deeper sense of empathy and compassion for others. We begin to see the world through a lens of abundance rather than scarcity, recognizing the ways in which we can make a difference, no matter how small our actions may seem.

By embracing the power of generosity, we open our hearts to the beauty of human connection and the joy that comes from giving. Let's continue to spread kindness and compassion wherever we go, knowing that our acts of generosity have the potential to create a more loving and caring world for all.

** Nurturing Your Soul Through Service**

Developing a sense of gratitude and humility can deepen your connection to the world around you. When you approach service with an open heart and a spirit of giving, you not only make a positive impact on others but also nourish your own soul. By recognizing the blessings in your life and being willing to share them with those in need, you tap into a wellspring of inner peace and joy.

Finding a balance between giving and receiving is essential in sustaining a meaningful service-oriented lifestyle. While it is important to offer your time, skills, and resources to others, it is equally crucial to allow yourself to receive help and support when needed. By embracing the cycle of giving and receiving, you create a harmonious flow of energy that enriches both your life and the lives of those around you.

Creating lasting impact through service-oriented living involves making intentional choices that align with your values and beliefs. Whether you volunteer regularly, donate to charitable causes, or simply show kindness and compassion in your daily interactions, every act of service has the potential to ripple out and create positive change in the world. By nurturing your soul through service, you not only contribute to the greater good but also nurture your own sense of purpose and fulfillment.

"See how the masses of men worry themselves into nameless graves; while here and there a great, unselfish soul forgets himself into mortality."

–Unknown

11

Conclusion

Hopefully, you have discovered that invincible health is a very holistic pursuit. There is an indisputable mind-body-spirit connection. We must nurture each of these aspects of our being if we are to experience life to its fullest. Quantum physicists are coming to believe that the universe operates in the realm of energy frequencies. Therefore, anything we can do to increase the vibrational frequency of our thoughts, and feelings along with the food and drink we consume will pay enormous dividends in terms of energy, vitality, and enthusiasm for life. The great Football Hall of Fame coach, Vince Lombardi noted; "Fatigue makes cowards of us all." Pay attention, be aware of, and choose carefully what you allow into your being for "a coward dies a thousand times, a brave man but once."; proclaimed some astute philosopher.

www.ingramcontent.com/pod-product-compliance
Lightning Source LLC
Chambersburg PA
CBHW051852250726
48659CB00006B/2173